Transform Your Body without Surgery

Valuable Insider Information to Painless Weight Loss and Physique Improvement

By: Maria Garcia

ISBN

PUBLISHERS NOTES

Disclaimer – Speedy Publishing LLC

This publication is intended to provide helpful and informative material. It is not intended to diagnose, treat, cure, or prevent any health problem or condition, nor is intended to replace the advice of a physician. No action should be taken solely on the contents of this book. Always consult your physician or qualified health-care professional on any matters regarding your health and before adopting any suggestions in this book or drawing inferences from it.

The author and publisher specifically disclaim all responsibility for any liability, loss or risk, personal or otherwise, which is incurred as a consequence, directly or indirectly, from the use or application of any contents of this book.

Any and all product names referenced within this book are the trademarks of their respective owners. None of these owners have sponsored, authorized, endorsed, or approved this book.

Always read all information provided by the manufacturers' product labels before using their products. The author and publisher are not responsible for claims made by manufacturers.

This book was originally printed before 2014. This is an adapted reprint by Speedy Publishing LLC with newly updated content designed to help readers with much more accurate and timely information and data.

Speedy Publishing LLC

40 E Main Street, Newark, Delaware, 19711

Contact Us: 1-888-248-4521

Website: http://www.speedypublishing.co

REPRINTED Paperback Edition: ISBN:

Manufactured in the United States of America

DEDICATION

This book is dedicated to my father, Anton. I grew up looking up to you. That's not going to change anytime soon. I love you, dad.

TABLE OF CONTENTS

Chapter 1 - What is Bodyweight Training?

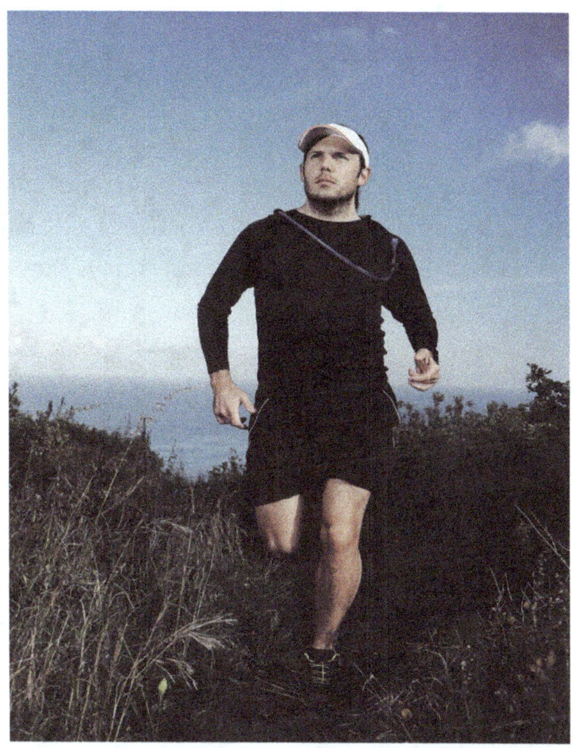

Fitness and strength building trends can be a dime a dozen. Those of us who have had a glimpse behind the fitness industry scenes have often seen firsthand what motivates its gurus. It is not how to help people get fit, fast or experience vibrant health, but how to shovel more cash into their bank accounts.

What if there were a proven fitness method, that didn't require any special equipment, no gym membership or supplement and diet options were strictly your own decision? This would be bad news for the health and fitness profiteers and great news for you wouldn't it?

Welcome to Bodyweight Training.

This method holds all these qualities and more. By the time you are through with this guide you will have all the information you need to build a new ripped and powerful you and you can do it all in your living room or backyard!

The History of Bodyweight Training

The inarguable fact is that no other strength and conditioning method has such a shining history of effectiveness. Going all the way back to ancient times and lasting until today. Don't take my word for it.

Here are some historical highlights of Bodyweight Training:

• The Indian Wrestling Cults

Did you know Indian wrestling as a sport (and near religion) goes back thousands of years? Approaching modern MMA in its mix of grappling and striking, Indian wrestlers developed extensive libraries of Bodyweight Training exercises, some revived in the last decade or so outside of India like the Hindu pushup and Hindu squat. The physical prowess of Indian wrestlers is legendary with well documented programs that included over 500 push ups and 1000 squats a day, six days a week!

• The Spartan Warriors

If you've ever seen a statue or painting of a Spartan warrior you will probably have seen that the movie "300" was right on the mark with their depiction of the Spartan physique. The Spartans lifted no weights, but trained using advanced Bodyweight Training methods which left them with a still lasting reputation of being some of the finest physical specimen to ever walk the earth.

- The Roman Gladiator

A distant cousin of the Spartan, Roman Gladiators employed similar training programs brought to them from the Greeks. Their results were equally impressive.

- Charles Atlas and the American Physical Culturalists

The idea of building a healthy, great looking and powerful body first reignited in modern days at the start of the 1900's. Probably the most popular and well known of these fitness enthusiasts was the legendary Charles Atlas. Charles, along with most of his contemporaries, was dedicated Bodyweight Training advocates and built insanely well developed and athletically capable bodies. Google Charles Atlas, Earle Liederman, Jack Lalanne or other fitness gurus of their era and marvel at what they were able to achieve minus weights, anabolic steroids, supplements or even advanced diet ideas!

- Modern Military Spec Ops

From the American Navy Seals to the British RAF and every Special Forces group in between has been built on a foundation of push-ups, pull ups, crunches and so on. Very few indulge in much weight training. Can anyone really deny their high level of conditioning and life and death level of true functional fitness?

- Matt Furey and the New Breed of Bodyweight Training

In the early 2000's a somewhat over the top fitness coach and author is credited by most as bringing back Bodyweight Training to the forefront of discussion and reviving a whole arsenal of lost exercises. Furey opened these doors and deserves more credit than he sometimes receives.

Now it should be clear you are about to follow in some very legendary footsteps when you dive into Bodyweight Training. Are you ready to carry on this proud fitness tradition? I think you absolutely have what it takes. Time to move forward!

Benefits of Weight Training

1. Lift Weights and Burn Calories 24 / 7. When you do even light weight training three to five days a week your body responds by amping up your metabolism twenty four hours a day, seven days a week!

2. Get More Confidence as You Get Stronger. There's something really magical about the confidence that comes along with getting stronger. Nothing positively adjusts a person's self-image like seeing himself become more powerful from weight training. This carries over to all areas of life and will be nothing, but a huge boost in your efforts to slim down!

3. Lifting Weights Slows Aging. Studies have shown resistance training dramatically slows down the aging process. That goes a long way as you strive to build a new slim, better looking and better feeling you doesn't it? This positive effect covers not only things like your skin, but even helps keep your bones young, strong and healthy!

Chapter 2- How to Build Upper Body Muscle Power

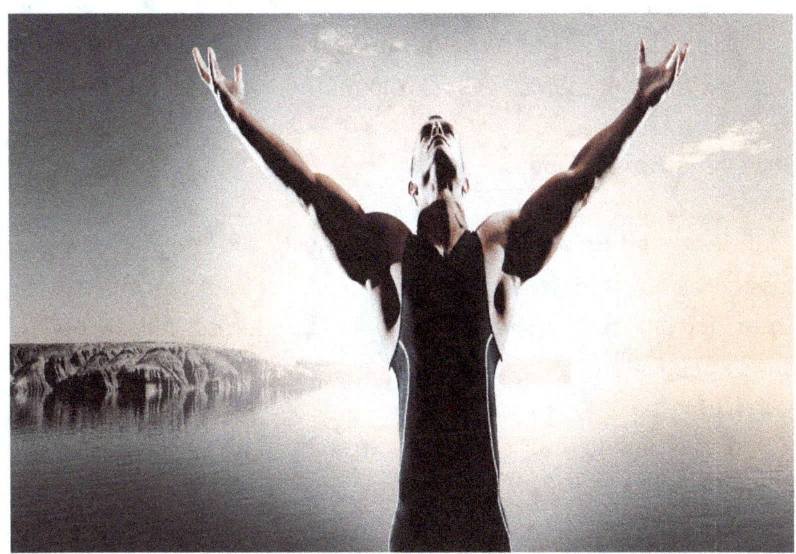

No matter what type of training we engage in safety should always come first. Bodyweight training is no exception to this golden rule. After all when injured we can hardly train at all can we? So paying close attention to things like warming up and stretching before our training sessions ultimately leads us to getting stronger and fitter in no time at all.

Bodyweight Training Warm Ups

Warming up for Bodyweight Training is much less complicated than some of the schemes you may be used to if you have done much weight lifting. Our goal is to get the blood flowing and raise our temperature before we do our light stretching. This helps make us more limber for our stretches and further reduces our chance of injury.

How you choose to do this is really a matter of personal choice, but I suggest you aim for the ten minute mark. A brisk walk or jog is what I choose to do most often, but if you prefer using the bike or a rowing machine that's fine too. Many of my friends who are involved in combat sports go old school and jump rope or hit the punching heavy bag. As long as we accomplish the goal of getting our blood circulating and temperature rising without overdoing it feel free to choose which ever cardio method you prefer.

Stretching Tips and Ideas

Again warming up and stretching is a must before every workout session. After your ten minute warm up another ten minutes of stretching unless you have special needs to address will get the job done effectively.

- Don't Bounce in Your Stretches. Stretch calmly and with a slow and controlled effort. This will not only give you the best results, but all will avoid tearing any tight muscles. We are stretching to prevent injury NOT cause injury!

- Control Your Breathing. Erratic breathing can detract from the benefits of stretching. Exhale into your stretch and continue breathing full deep breaths as you maintain your stretch.

- The Magic Thirty. Hold your stretches for thirty seconds. Research has shown this is the amount of time that offers the most benefit for the athlete.

- Never Stretch into Pain. Stretching should NOT hurt. "No pain - no gain" may apply to other areas of training. It never, ever applies to stretching! Please don't ignore this tip.

- Consider having a go at Yoga. Yoga can be a really awesome compliment to Bodyweight Training. The false impression that yoga is just for women is losing more ground every day, with

Football and Rugby players, along with mixed martial artists all singing the praises of this ancient art form. Yoga can help you experience real health benefits along with flexibility. Combined with Bodyweight Training you can truly build the ideal body in the privacy of your own home with no equipment needed at all.

Between warming up and stretching you'll be ready to train in twenty minutes. Give these twenty minutes the same attention you pay to the rest of your training and your body will thank you. It goes a long way towards becoming near injury proof!

The Pushups and Dips

A solid hard chest, horse shoe triceps and ripped abs too. Sky rocketing upper body power. Even bragging rights among friends. The pushup and its cousin the bodyweight dip offer all this and much more. If you had to choose only two exercises to perform this would be the first half (the second being pull ups of course!) Exploring the Pushup

Used everywhere from the school yard, to the gym and dojo to the sand and dirt of special forces training camps the push up is rightly beloved as one of the simplest and best exercises we could ever perform. Embrace it.

Here are some pushup tips to keep in mind.

• Always use Proper Pushup Form.

Many of us have picked up bad habits in the way we execute our pushups over the years. Here's proper pushup form:

1. Keep yourself stiff and tight - including your abs.

2. Elbows at a forty five degree angle at the sides of your body.

3. Take a breath as you lower your chest to the floor.

4. Exhale as you press up.

5. Repeat.

• Engage your Mind while doing Pushups.

It's helpful to visualize your palms exploding through the floor while doing your pushups as a means to building more explosive power.

• Raise your Feet for an Upper Chest Emphasis

Place your feet on a chair, bed or better yet an inflatable exercise ball to focus the emphasis of the pushup more greatly on the upper chest and shoulders. This can help develop a more pleasing physique by most accounts.

• Don't Be Frightened to Go High Volume

It's not uncommon for Bodyweight Training enthusiasts to do 100, 250 or even 500 pushups every few days. Ignore those who cry about "over training" from Bodyweight training. This has proven to give fantastic results and is exactly the method used in modern military - and in prisons too, to build seriously hard and strong muscle!

Dynamic Dipping

After pushups our next powerful chest, triceps and really total upper body builder is the dip. How we choose to do dips depends on our strength levels, conditioning and what we have in our surroundings to perform our dips on.

• Parallel Bar Dips.

This is the traditional dip that requires the most starting strength to begin training with. With your hands on two bars (or handles) you dip your entire body and press it back up using your upper body power. Many school yards have parallel bars to dip from allowing you to train for free in the sun while forging a mighty upper body.

• Chair Dips.

Putting your hands on a chair behind your back while your legs are extended and heels resting on a second chair (your body should be roughly "L" shaped) this offers a much easier dip version for those who find full dips too difficult.

• The Atlas Dip.

This is my personal favorite of the dips taken from the Golden Age strong man and physical culture guru Charles Atlas. Two chairs are placed in front of you about 20 inches apart depending on how wide your shoulders are. Place a hand on each chair seat while your body is extended behind you, feet on the floor. Perform pushups between the chairs. Atlas suggested way back in 1922 for his students to do at least 200 a day, working their way up to what he did - 500! This is a really superb exercise many modern trainers aren't aware of. It can be a game changer in building a great looking chest, shoulders and triceps too! Try it and I think you will be impressed with your results.

With this information rejoice! A new chest is now right around the corner!

Pull Ups

You should not consider yourself anywhere near being strong, fit or in shape if you can't do a pull up. Thanks to the modern age of "all show - no go" fitness machines we've had at least a generation of trainers doing everything they can to avoid hitting the pull up bar. Pull downs, back machines, bands, on and on and on trying to "fix" an exercise that was never broke in the first place. We all know not to fix things that aren't broke don't we? If not we certainly should!

With that behind us many may start their Bodyweight Training journey with the need to build strength and power in their pull up ability. This will reap tremendous benefits - the more pull ups you do regularly the better you will look and feel. Ninety days of pull ups will likely leave you looking like an action movie star or superhero.

Follow these suggestions and you'll be doing sets of twenty in no time!

• Avoid Going to Failure.

In building Pull Up strength and power it's been shown again and again it's best to avoid going to failure in sets. Always leave a rep or two in the bank. Do more sets while avoiding going to failure rather than blowing out all your energy on only one or two sets. Even though this may seem counter initiatory this will quickly turn into huge jumps in strength. Olympic athletes swear by this method. Try it and you will too!

• Pull With the Lats First.

Pull with your back muscles first NOT with your arms. Obviously your lats being much larger muscles they possess more power and endurance than your biceps. Use this to your advantage.

• Keep Your Elbows Pointing Back and Down.

These will aide you in firing your lats in the movement. Try to image elbowing someone behind you in their stomach. Like the guy who convinced you to add this grueling exercise to your Bodyweight training sessions (just kidding!)

• Get your Chin over the Bar.

There's no need to go chest to the bar like some trainers claim. Anything much beyond your chin does little to add further to your back development. Instead consider your chin going over the bar as a good solid rep.

• Lose Body Fat.

The leaner you are the better your pull up ability will become. Fat people don't do many pull ups and pull up masters are very rarely (if ever) fat. When you set a goal of putting up massive numbers on the pull up bar, it's a good sign of encouragement in the quest to also get lean. One drive compliments the other quite nicely!

• Switch Up Your Grips.

Okay technically speaking pull ups are when your palms are facing you. Chin ups are when your palms are facing away from you. Neutral grips are when you are using a bar that allows your palms to be facing each other. Do a few sets of each when you train upper body. This will help build your back from different angles and also do wonders for your grip strength!

There's no better feeling than being able to hop up and grab the bar pounding out easy reps of pull ups. It's a lost art even the big and strong in bodybuilding gyms are usually unable to manage. Put in smart and steady work and you'll be leaving jaws open and fielding questions on how you built up your new found pull up power! Feel free to tell them about our guide.

CHAPTER 3- HOW TO BUILD LOWER BODY MUSCLE POWER

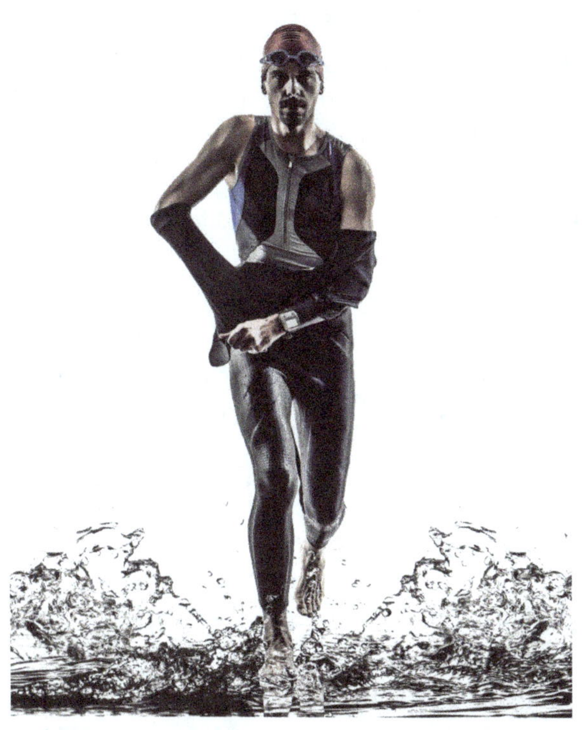

You may have heard one of the ignorant claims that it's impossible to build powerful and aesthetically pleasing looking legs without throwing half a ton on the leg press machine or squatting 500lbs. Never mind what that type of non-stop pounding often ends up doing to the knees. Ask anyone who has power lifted or follow exclusively heavy bodybuilding leg routines for over ten years if you don't believe me. I guarantee many mention a knee surgery or two.

The great news is that legs respond exceptionally well to high rep training Bodyweight methods. Size, strength, endurance and shapeliness are all within reach doing the following bodyweight exercises alone. You will also be much more likely to stay injury free! Can't beat that can you?

• Bodyweight Squat.

This is the foundation of your Bodyweight leg training routine. Lock your fingers behind your head and drop glutes to the floor. Explode up. Repeat. Also called prisoner squats for their popularity behind bars these will build true explosive leg power, flexibility and endurance too. Aim for a few hundred a session. A close friend uses these as his full cardio workout and twenty to thirty minutes of Bodyweight Squats a day has left him ripped to the bone! This is cooler than running on a treadmill that's for sure.

• Bodyweight Lunges.

Lunge forward with one going as low as possible. The knee of your rear leg should come close to touching the floor. Step back to standing and repeat with opposite leg. This is a good secondary movement to the Bodyweight Squat that can strengthen your glutes and cut up your quads even further.

• Toe Raises.

Stand on stairs or box with one leg. Rise up on tip of your toes engaging your calf muscle. Drop down as far as possible. Repeat. When finished switch legs and do the same amount of reps. Excellent calf builder where you should aim for as many reps as possible.

• Jumping Jacks.

I'm sure you remember these as a kid don't you? Use jumping jacks as both a leg builder and cardio tool. Rather than reps, set an alarm clock for a certain time and try to beat it at each session. Don't be surprised when your body fat quickly melts away as your lower body gets more toned and stronger. Those old gym teachers in physical education class seem to have had much more actionable knowledge than they often are given credit for... further proof that in the field of strength and conditioning newer is not always better. Sometimes falling back on old near forgotten methods represents the true cutting edge in building a new and better body!

All in all see for yourself what a great leg workout you can get using a few fairly simple exercises, focused with power and intensity while never touching a weight or stepping on a machine. After you do, try your best not to laugh in the face of the next person sweating on the Stair Master or doing 150lb leg extensions. Once you are in on this secret and powerful fitness knowledge I can tell you it's definitely tempting! But don't forget we all have to start somewhere!

Chapter 4- Building the Neck, Back and Core Muscles

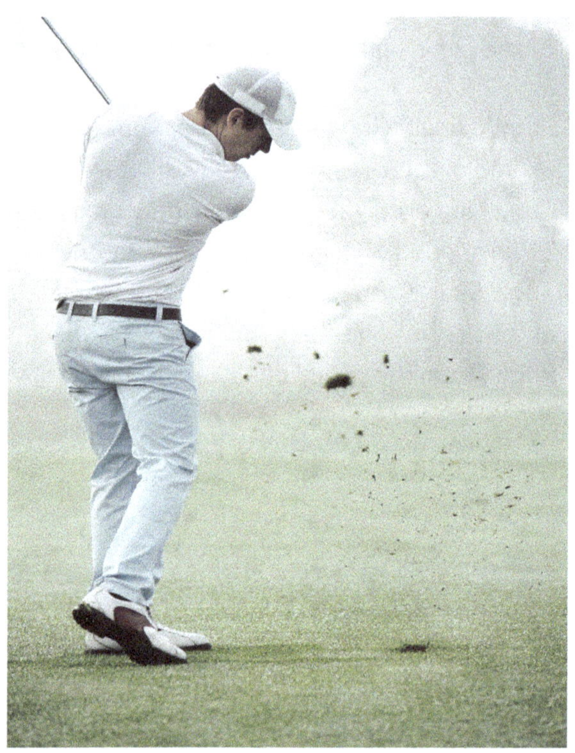

It may not be the first thing people check out when you sun tan on the beach, but a strong lower back can save you all sorts of headaches in life. From making you less injury prone at work or protecting the spine if you engage in any hard contact sports, time spent training the lower back can be rightly thought of very much as a health insurance policy in all the best ways.

A Bodyweight Exercise from the wrestler's tool box - the Back and Neck Bridge offer us the best of the best lower back builders, once again completely ignored by mainstream trainers and fitness gurus. Never use one of those dumb back extension machines ever again!

Here are some thoughts concerning the Wrestler's Bridge...

• Try to Get a First Hand Lesson in Bridging.

It's important before you try to do your first back bridge to ideally get a lesson from someone with bridging experience face to face. If this isn't possible take the tips from this guide, read a bit further on the internet and watch some of the many YouTube demonstrations before you try your first go at it. When done correctly they are more than safe, but having a clear visual lesson on the proper technique is a must just to be sure no mistakes are made.

• Start with Wall Walks.

Stand with your back to a wall roughly two feet away. Arch your back and slowly and securely wall walk down with your hands continuing to arch your back. This will condition your lower back for full floor wrestler's bridges in a short time.

• Back Bridge Details

The wrestler's back bridge is when you arch your back and your bodyweight is on your palms. Hold for time.

• Neck Bridge Details

The wrestler's neck bridge is when you arch your back and your bodyweight in on your forehead and neck. Also hold for time.

• Shoot for Duration NOT for Reps.

With bridging you are aiming to hold the bridge for longer and longer times at full extension, rather than working for reps. This builds tremendous strength, makes your stabilizer muscles powerful and even helps to develop supreme will power and force of mind. Using a small stop watch or kitchen timer is the best way to increase time under pressure without having to distract you counting.

• Always Stretch After Doing Bridges.

It's a great habit to get into doing "toe touch" leg stretches after back bridging to make sure you are conditioning both sides of your muscles as an injury prevention measure. Take around five minutes (or more if you'd like) to engage in stretching after your back and neck bridges.

• Skip if You Have Previous Back Injuries.

If you have prior lower back issues either skip the wrestler's bridges or get your Doctor's okay before you dive in. Remember safety always comes first!

Pushups pull ups, back bridges. Bodyweight Training is very much akin to old school fight training. It's real hard once you get momentum going to not feel like you're preparing for a prize fight and that's a great thing.

Our challenges may not be in a ring, but a fighting spirit and strong and healthy body makes all of life's obstacles much easier to overcome. I can tell you that much from hard earned personal experience!

How to Build a Core of Steel

Bodyweight Training has huge advantages over other training methodologies in many areas. The most shining of them is an area that's dear to nearly everyone interested in getting into great shape - developing a ripped and powerful core.

Let's be clear - no other style of training will give you six pack abs as quickly and with as extra little effort as Bodyweight Training.

Bodyweight Training is the perfect storm for getting the perfect core.

There are many reasons for this - first and foremost your abs and lower back are trained in nearly all of your major training movements. Pushups pull ups, Bodyweight squats - they all help build their target muscles groups while also as a bonus carve out your six pack. How's that for win / win?

Say good bye to the endless reps on the stupid abdominal crunch that never produced any results anyway. I doubt you'll miss it!

Here's a look at some Core Bodyweight Training exercises that shouldn't be neglected on your path to the abs of your dreams...

• The V Up.

Also called the "Atlas sit up." Lay on your back with your legs fully extended and curl your upper body up while also bringing up your legs. Touch finger tips to toes. This can be somewhat difficult if you are a bit out of shape - if so start with normal floor crunches and sit ups until a bit more core strength is developed. Just be sure to add the V ups as soon as possible they are more than worth the effort.

• Leg Raises.

Hanging from a pull up bar (which will also build your grip strength) raise your legs to an "L" position using your lower ab muscles. Beginners feel free to start by doing knee rather than full extended leg raises until more strength is built. Many fail to achieve a six or eight pack simply because they've neglected their lower abs.

• Plank. Lay in push up position.

Come up on elbows and forearms keeping your body straight tightening your abs as if you were about to be punched in the stomach. Hold for time - twenty seconds in a good start, working up to sets of sixty seconds or more.

• Side Plank.

This is perhaps the best overall exercise for building powerful oblique. Lie on your side and come up on your elbow keeping your body tight and in a straight line, tightening your core again as if preparing for a punch to the stomach. Hold for time.

• Mountain Climbers.

This is a powerful total body exercise with an emphasis on abs. It is also hugely effective as a cardio technique. Go into push up position. Press up and stay up. Alternate bringing knees to chest as quickly as possible. Go for time and expect to break a serious sweat. Mountain climbers are a true warrior's exercise - if you want a body that looks like something out of the movie 300 throws it all into your mountain climbers!

Ninety days of Bodyweight Training may well leave you with a bullet proof core - the type of abs no machine could ever produce. Let's do it!

CHAPTER 5- THE RIGHT DIET FOR BODY TRAINING

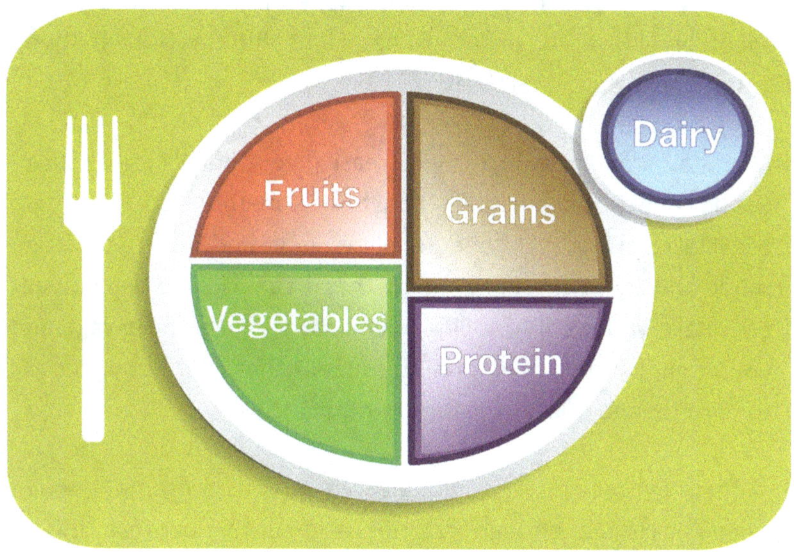

When losing weight, most individuals would skip eating breakfast thinking that it is an effective method of eliminating weight. Now, what they do not realize is that this technique is not really effective and could even cause negative effects on their bodies. When dieting, one of the most important things to be aware of is the importance of eating breakfast.

Breakfast is referred to "breakfast" simply because it breaks the long fast. People are asleep during the night for many hours, so in the morning, it is necessary to eat something in order to feel better and have the energy to face the new day. More importantly, having breakfast is vital to a fat burning diet. If you want to lose weight fast, be mindful to eat breakfast every day.

Here are some of the reasons and importance of eating breakfast to the body when dieting: • Breakfast will allow you to control your hunger and avoid eating snacks later on during the day. What would be the use of your diet when you would eventually eat more because you are hungry, since you skipped breakfast? If ever you skipped breakfast, just ensure to have a healthy snack so that you can still lose weight effectively.

• A healthy breakfast will aid in increasing your body's metabolism- Eating breakfast can actually boost one's metabolism. If you skip breakfast, you would tend to place your body into starvation mode and try to conserve energy that it can. Now, when you eat breakfast, you are also telling your body that you are awake and you are not fasting anymore. This means that your body is ready to burn fat and utilizes the energy during the day.

• A healthy breakfast would also help you consume enough calories- Having enough calories is essential because this is responsible in increasing your energy levels. When you regularly skip breakfast, you are also not consuming calories that would end up in dropping off of your energy levels. This would also slow down your metabolism. Losing weight would be that effective.

• Eating breakfast is essential in losing weight, as it helps the body attain its weight loss goal faster. According to research and studies, those individuals who miss breakfast are the ones who were 4 times more likely to be overweight. If you do not want to risk of gaining weight, ensure not to skip breakfast. These are some of the importance of eating breakfast to the body when dieting. Breakfast is the most essential meal of the day; therefore, it is necessary not to skip it. Of course, when dieting, just make sure that you follow a healthy breakfast so that you can efficiently lose weight and achieve your weight loss goals. Eating breakfast is good and healthy, so do not think that skipping breakfast would help you lose weight. This will just make you feel weak and unhealthy, and this will not do well with your goal of losing weight. Have a healthy breakfast every day and follow the right diet. In no time, you would be surprised to see the positive results with your health and body.

Hydrate

Drinking water plays a key role in dieting. If you ever find yourself stuck in a weight loss plateau despite following your diet program strictly, then it could be that you are not drinking enough water. Studies have shown that a lot people unsuspectingly suffer from severe or mild dehydration and you could be affected as well. Your body requires water for various biochemical processes.

The following are the benefits of drinking enough water to your body when dieting:

- Water assists the body in the conversion of fat reserves into energy. When the body is dehydrated, the body's metabolism processes are slowed down and this impedes the breakdown of fats in the body, and in effect, your weight loss. If this happens, your weight loss curve hits a plateau.

- Water holds naturally holds back your appetite. The hypothalamus region in your brain serves the role of controlling cravings and appetites, with the control centers for thirst and hunger situated next to one another. This means that drinking enough not only quenches your thirst, but it takes away the feelings of hunger as well. A study by Washington University found that drinking a glass of water before going to bed reduces mid-night cravings.

- Water also helps in the prevention of sagging skin which is a common side effect of weight loss. It gives the skin a healthier and youthful look by helping in the reconstruction of destroyed skin cells.

- Water assists in the elimination of waste products from the body. When dieting, the body loses weight and there are extra by products to be removed. This means that the body requires sufficient amounts of water into which the unwanted products will be dissolved and excreted from the body.

- Water is effective in dealing with constipation. If the body does not get enough water, it is compelled to siphon it from its internal reserves, normally the colon, resulting into constipation. Normal bowel function will resume once the body receives adequate water.

In general, mild dehydration leads to a number of health complications. Mild dehydration is characterized by the following symptoms: fatigue, cravings, headaches and constipation. However, as soon as you get the water in balance, you achieve what diet experts refer to as a breakthrough point. At this point, as fluid retention in the body eases, the liver and endocrine systems start to operate more effectively, helping to reinstate your natural thirst, while reducing your cravings significantly. This eventually results into heightened metabolism rates which facilitate the breakdown and loss of fat in the body.

How Much Water Does the Body Need?

In conclusion, the above benefits clearly show the importance of drinking water, particularly if you are on a diet. Nonetheless, everyone should make drinking water a habit. It should not only be done when you are thirsty as thirst, in itself, is an indication of the presence of dehydration. Hence, every adult ought to take at least eight glasses of water every day during cold weather. Since there is a lot of perspiration and loss of liquid during hot weather, additional glasses of water must be taken.

Lastly, if exercises are part of your dieting plan, ensure that you drink 6-12 ounces of fluids after 15-20 intervals. This way, you will maintain the most favorable fluid balance during your exercises

How to Shop Right to Eat Better

It's a bit shocking how many people attempt to follow a healthy fat burning diet and exercise program without investing the time into understanding how to read nutrition labels on food products. Not knowing what's in the food you eat makes slimming down a near impossible task. On the flip side, once you understand food labels you can shop better, to eat better.

Let's take a look at what they reveal so we can make wiser diet choices.

• Serving Size.

Please pay complete and total attention to this number. Everything that follows will apply to only 1 serving. Unscrupulous food companies will often exaggerate the number of servings in a container or package to make it seem the calorie count is lower. Don't fall for this devious diet destroying trick!

• Percentage of Daily Value.

This is based on a 2000 calorie a day diet for a moderately active person. Use it only as a rough guideline as it can vary greatly based on gender, activity level, age, height, weight and so on.

- Calories. Pretty self-explanatory this is the total number of calories contained per serving.

- Fat

This is further broken down into saturated fats, Trans fat, Monounsaturated and Polyunsaturated fats. Both saturated and Trans fat should be avoided. Monounsaturated and Polyunsaturated fats, on the other hand carry some health benefits. These are the healthier fats found in things like olive oil and avocado.

- Cholesterol

Doctors suggest keeping your cholesterol intake below 300mgs a day to avoid the risk of heart disease. Below 150mgs a day is an even better target.

- Sodium.

High sodium intake will make you retain water and weigh more on the scale. For a healthy heart it's suggested to stay below 1500mgs a day. Keep an eye on prepared food they are often over loaded with sodium!

- Carbohydrates.

Split between fiber (very good) and sugar (very bad). Aim for a low carb intake while slimming down and things will go much, much smoother.

• Protein.

Treat this as your best friend. Aim for around .5 a gram for every pound you weigh. If you are working out very hard more is even better. This is where most of your calories should be coming from.

• Vitamins and Minerals.

This includes the vitamins and minerals naturally contained in the food as well as anything artificially added by the manufacturer.

• Ingredients.

These will be listed in order of the amount contained in the food product. Here's another area where some companies will try to deceive so pay close attention!

Now you are fully armed with the information needed to be able to shop smart and be able to understand the nutrition labels on food products. While slimming down, like in a great many other areas of life, knowledge is power. How does it feel to have power over your food choices? Good I hope. It will serve you well.

Chapter 6- Macronutrients Matter

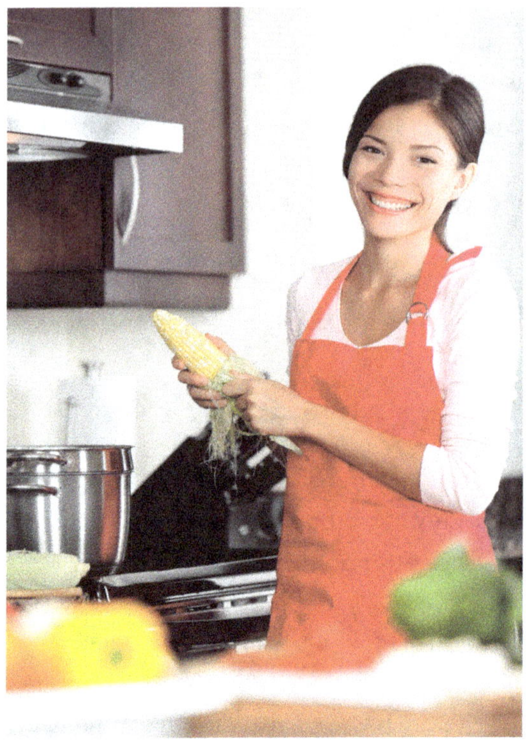

For our weight loss purposes we can view our diets as basically being split between two important categories. The first is micronutrients - which includes vitamins and minerals, things we need in small quantities that don't carry calories. Most of us are quite familiar with the ins and outs of micronutrients.

Much more vital for our weight loss success is the second category of macronutrients - protein, carbohydrates and fats. These three things we require in large amounts to function and how we manipulate them can mean the difference between success and failure!

Let's look at all three macronutrients.

• Protein.

Protein is the building block of our new lean bodies, absolutely essential to help us look and feel great and to speed up our recovery from hard work out sessions. Keeping our protein levels high will also bring us lots of other benefits - even keeping us more resistant to things like the common cold. It's worth repeating we should aim for .5 a gram of protein for every pound we weigh while slimming down. Here are some common protein counts of food you may enjoy: a 4 oz chicken breast has 36 grams of protein, a whole egg has 6 grams of protein, a glass of milk 16 grams and most protein shakes 28 grams of protein a serving. If your protein levels are consistently low you can expect slower strength gains, fatigue and possibly even injury!

• Carbohydrates.

Carbohydrates are the main source of energy in our diets. While a requirement for even dieters to function efficiently, over indulgence in carbohydrates has been the death blow of many a weight loss plan.

A smart level of carbohydrates to start off with before tweaking your diet is right around 30% of your daily calories (the rest split between protein and healthy fats). This should be slowly lowered if you are having difficulties shedding body fat. Sugary carbs and things like white rice, white pasta and potatoes should be eaten infrequently, if at all.

• Fats.

Let's clear up one of the most common diet misconceptions, once and for all. All fats do NOT make you fat. In fact many are health and weight loss miracle workers. Flax seed oil, fish oil and to a lesser degree unsaturated fats like olive oil are all important parts of your diet. Try to take in about 3 grams of flax or fish oil a day and be prepared to both see yourself lose weight faster as your metabolism increases and your overall quality of life improve as well. Inflammation will decrease, your skin and hair will look great and many guys will also see marked increases in their sex drive! There's hardly any other addition you could make to your diet that is quite so transformative!

Do you feel like you have a better understanding of macronutrients? These easy to follow tips will quickly have them working in your Slim Down favor. Dieting can be effective without getting anywhere near being complicated.

CHAPTER 7- THE IMPORTANCE OF PROPER SLEEP AND RECOVERY

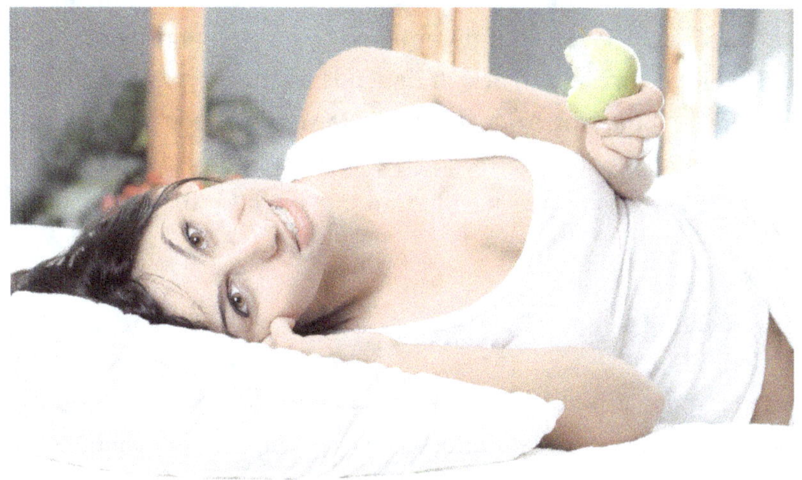

To consider sleep as an activity is difficult. One assumes sleep to be a phase of inactivity or rest. But, the matter of fact is, that sleep is that active phase in our entire day's routine, when numerous bodily functions are expedited. The sales data of sleep inducing tranquilizers and sleeping pills prove the rising cases of sleep deficiency that owes a lot to the modern lifestyle. While profound research is available on the importance of exercise for the body, few embark on the desire to learn about rest and sleep...yet it is one of the most important factors in overall health and well-being.

What Is Sleep?

Firstly, it's important to understand that while the body rests, the mind and the brain go on a restorative hyper-drive. Bodily signals are sent to the various organs of to begin its build up for the next hour of optimum action. The more sleep deprived a person is, the more the chances of deficient physical and mental activity, as you've not allowed your body to recover from the previous bout or prepare for the next. Sleep is a period of nerve and muscle relaxation which begins a period of repair and rejuvenation of all the tissues and organs, much needed after a day of hectic often strenuous activity. Sleep is determined by a certain biological cycle called as the 'circadian clock'. It depends on the intervals of certain number of hours of being awake followed by sleep, and so on. Other elements affecting it could be- the amount of light, stress levels, metabolism levels and even the medication we may be taking.

The Power of Sleep

Sleep is a powerful energy booster owing to the fact that while we sleep the process called 'anabolism' gets underway; understood more simply as the recovery process for cells and tissues through the production of enzymes and proteins. It in fact counteracts the effect of 'catabolism' or the process that occurs as you exercise or work- out during the day which produces an action wherein energy is released from cells. This affects the molecular components of the body. If your catabolism exceeds anabolism, little growth will happen. Thus those who strain themselves with a tougher workout or play an extra hour must give their body the extra rest to sustain their growth of muscle mass, which is directly proportionate to fitness.

There is no contention to the fact that mental alertness, concentration levels, communication, creativity, emotional balance and the productivity levels of an individual is also affected by the amount of sleep.

Prolonged sleep deprivation has been linked to anxiety and depression. Sleep induces the release of certain hormones that affect the central nervous system of the body thus affecting mood and emotional stability. Less sleep increases Cortisol which is a catabolic hormone and it decreases testosterone levels that are directly related to muscle mass gain. Less sleep also means a higher insulin level that increases your body's resistance to nutritional absorption.

While one cannot contest the importance of fitness training including weight training one must understand the mechanics of what really happens to the body while this physical stress is being faced. While we exercise or lift weights, the muscle contracts or crunches thereby getting compressed or shortened.

This happens when the muscle microfibers compress. With every stimulus you give to your body, the muscle is strained to respond. What must however be realized is that between the phases of stimulus, the muscle needs to recover from it by building new bridges across the new muscle groups that are slowly forming. This growth is only possible when the body rests.

Another disturbing consequence that comes with compromising on the amount of sleep has is in the raised levels of cortisone which has been directly linked to more abdominal fats .While there has been encyclopedic quantum of research on the benefits of fitness programs, very little attention is paid to the importance of the body and its sleep requirement.

Balancing heavy workouts with its milder versions and adequate breaks from strenuous routines is not only the best antidote for perfect health; it's the best way to gain optimal benefits from your exercise routine.

CHAPTER 8- THE WONDERS OF RESISTANCE TRAINING

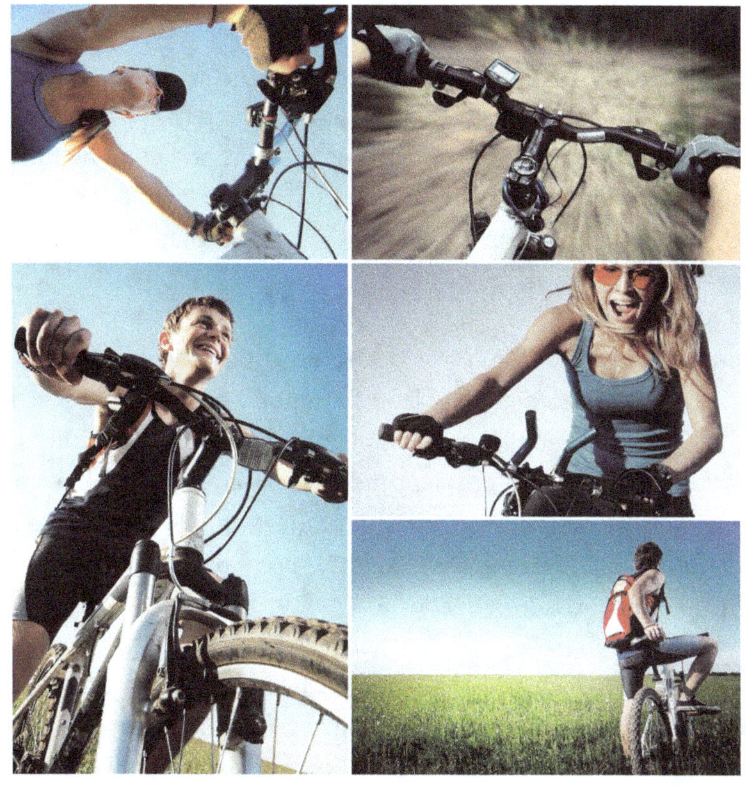

Excess weight is one of the most common problems that affect very many people from all across the globe. There is need to lose this unwanted weight so as to avoid health complications such as heart attack and other related diseases.

Below is a detailed guide of the importance of resistance training for losing weight.

Increase metabolic rate- The Wetabolic rate refers to the rate at which the body converts fats into energy for various purposes. Resistance training helps to increase the rate at which the fats are metabolized and this in turn helps to significantly reduce body fat.

Improves Body Posture- Since virtually all the physical activities in this category involves all the body muscles, they help to strengthen and increase muscles. This in turn helps one to improve body posture.

Increase Blood Circulation- For the body organs to operate optimally, they have to have sufficient and uninterrupted supply of blood rich in various nutrients such as proteins and carbohydrates. Resistance training helps to ensure that blood circulation in the body is optimal. This in turn helps to ensure that all vital body organs operate normally.

Decreases the Risk of Injuries- Losing weight involves a number of physical activities which may lead to injuries especially during the first stages. For example, new members might experience joint and muscles pains but this problem fades away as the body becomes acquainted to the activity. Resistance training will help decrease your susceptibility to injuries since the body parts will be able to withstand the pressure effectively.

Prevent cardiovascular diseases as well as Arthritis and diabetes- Excess weight has being closely linked to a number of health complications. Due to fact that these exercises will reduce and prevent accumulation of fats in the body, your chances of suffering from various cardiovascular diseases, diabetes and arthritis will be reduced significantly.

Boost Self Esteem- In most cases, persons suffering from excess weight problem are often stigmatized by the society. Fortunately, resistance training will help reduce this stigmatization and boost your self-esteem.

Improves your Sleep Patterns- Excess weight can distort your sleeping pattern especially if the issue is stressing you too much.

Through these physical activities, you will be able to solve this problem completely. This will in turn help you sleep much better at night as well as boost your productivity at home or at your work place.

Increase Bone Density and Strength- As the name suggest, this training will not only help you lose weight but also increase your bone density and strength. Increased bone strength will help reduce your susceptibility to injuries as well as enhance your performance of various physical tasks.

Be sure to consult a professional medical practitioner before enrolling in a particular program so as to avoid any health complications. Last but not least, ensure that your follow the instructions given by your trainer so as to achieve the full benefits from this training.

Myths about Resistance Training

1. Women who do strength training will become bulky and muscular

This myth has been around for so many years and unfortunately a lot of women believe it. Women do not have the ability to bulk up when they do resistance training exercises to increase their metabolism. Those who bulk up are the ones that take male hormones and inject anabolic steroids into their body. These kinds of women are mostly professional body builders. Therefore if you want to achieve that bulky look, it is very clear what you have to do. However, if you just want to achieve a lean toned body, resistance training exercises will give you just that; no bulky shoulders or arms.

2. Weights and expensive gym equipment are necessary for resistance training exercises

While free weights and other gym equipment are necessary to speed up your progress, they are not necessarily the only things that you can use to build muscles. There are a variety of ways that you can build muscle and some of them include: resistance bands, bar method, Pilate's, using your own body weight and isometric training. There are many programs for resistance training that do not use any equipment yet they help people to achieve excellent results.

3. When you grow old you cannot build muscle

This is not true because studies show that even people who are 70 years old can build muscle. In addition, people who are in their 50's or even 40's can be able to build adequate muscle mass with just a few training sessions per week.

4. Resistance training requires hours and hours of training per day

This takes the crown for being the biggest misconception about resistance training that can help boost your metabolism. Experts believe that as long as you eat a healthy well balanced diet and you do not have any diseases, you will only need about 20 minutes to half an hour sessions per week for you to realize results.

It is not the hours that you spend at the gym training but it is how often you do them and how hard you push your body. It has been established that when you add even a pound of muscle, your metabolism will increase and you can burn up to a maximum of 50 calories per day.

Imagine how many calories you can burn when you add 10 pounds of muscle.

5. You will need to constantly lift heavy weights in order to maintain muscle mass

If you train every day you are likely to build more muscle and speed up your metabolism, right? Wrong! It has been proven that the people who achieve phenomenal results are the ones that take breaks in between their work out days. Muscles are built when our bodies are resting and not when they are active as most people would like to believe. The body also needs to recover after an intense work-out session.

Chapter 9 - Body Transformation is a Lifestyle

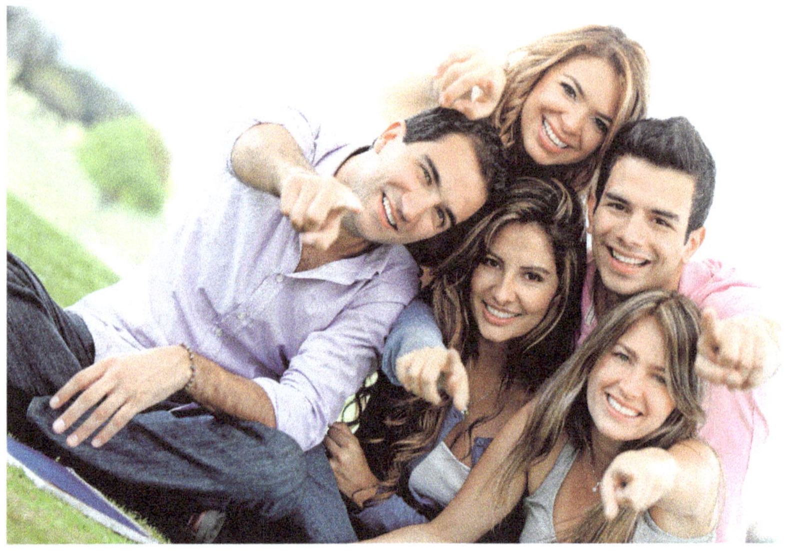

Whenever a special occasion or a holiday draws near, people often scramble for quick weight loss products or programs. While looking good in swimwear during summer is not a bad idea, looking for a short cut to weight loss can backfire. Truth is weight loss is a lifestyle and not a fad. It is a result of a consistent effort that involves exercise, proper food intake, and the right amount of rest. This key will reveal how to achieve a healthy lifestyle that helps shed pounds permanently.

First, you have to change your perception about weight loss. It's not just a matter of watching your weight on the scale. Weight loss should be about changing your body composition by having less body fat and acquiring more muscles. For women, this means losing side handles and toning your thighs. For men, it mainly means decreasing your waist line. Lately, health experts are associating heart disease risks with a large waistline. Hence, having ripped abs is not just for aesthetic reasons but mainly for longevity.

Maria Garcia

Weight loss is a goal to achieve good health; looking good should only be a consequence.

Second, you have to exercise on a daily basis if possible.

Start with brisk walking if you're overweight to prevent knee injuries. Perform this activity consistently by spending at least twenty minutes a day. Or, you can try a high intensity interval training (HIIT) to jumpstart your metabolism. Samples of which are burpees, body squats, push-ups, and mountain climbers. This is way shorter to perform but requires cardiovascular health and lower body weight. It shocks the body to drastically increase metabolism that results to weight loss. However, this is not advisable for people who are just beginning to exercise.

Third, educate yourself on proper food intake. People who need to lose weight should consume less than their total energy expenditure. Plus, macronutrients like protein take center stage along with complex carbohydrates. Reducing consumption of sugary food products does a lot of good to your body. Hyperlidimia, a condition where the body has high levels of cholesterol, is often triggered by obesity and diabetes.

Avoid eating fast-food. Prepare meals and bring them to work. Choose lean ground meat and season them with spices. Then, make sure you have a side dish of vegetables to add more fiber in your diet.

Lastly, minimize stress in your life by managing them. Again, you can resort to exercise to shake off stress from work. Listen to relaxing music. Enjoy time with your family or pursue a hobby you love. Stress produces hormones like cortisol that sabotage our attempts at weight loss. Also, get enough sleep so your mind and body can function optimally.

As you can see, weight loss is a lifestyle and not a fad. It means prioritizing exercise over a sedentary lifestyle. It means choosing the right food to fuel your body. Most of all, it means a healthy perspective of what life is all about - taking care of yourself for your loved ones

Transform Your Body Today!

Exercise

It's the surest and most natural way to lose weight. Exercising can be done in so many ways to fit into your daily activities. For instance, you can decide to cycle to and from your work place or shopping center instead of taking a bus. On the other hand, you can opt to use the stairs instead of the elevator. Other activities like walking, jogging and running will also contribute to weight loss.

You can make exercising fun too, like playing basketball with your peers or kids, going on long walks with your loved ones and many more fun activities that eventually will burn calories. On the other hand, you can structure an exercising routine every day that will involve at least 30 minutes of cardiovascular exercises.

Remember, exercises on top of burning up fat and calories also help in building a lean muscles mass which is essential for the body's metabolic rate.

Consume the Right Drinks

If it's not possible to quit alcohol entirely, limit yourself to a maximum of two on isolated cases when you have to take alcohol. Alcohol has no nutritional value to the body and the body usually uses it as its first energy source. Eventually, the food consumed ends up being stored as fat in the body. Alcohol also influences you to eat the wrong type of foods, preferably junk foods that are high in calories. It's, therefore, essential to avoid alcohol consumption, or to limit its consumption, as much as possible.

Similarly, avoid fruit drinks and soda. Instead opt for diet drinks and plenty of water. Water suppresses the regular urges to eat and consequently help you lose some weight. It also keeps the body hydrated, which is ideal for nutrients' release to the body.

Green tea is also favorite beverage for people on a weight loss program. Studies have demonstrated that consuming green tea leads to more calories being burnt faster than those who do not consume it.

Consume the Right Foods

Eat the right foods that will not contribute to weight gain but rather to weight loss. Grape fruit has been found effective in helping people lose weight. Consuming half a grape fruit three times a day burns more calories by boosting the body's metabolism.

On the other hand, avoid or minimize on the consumption of fats, especially animal fats as they are high in cholesterol. Opt for skim milk and low fat cheese. Similarly, consume lean meat, preferably white meat. In addition, opt for unprocessed foods as their calories and fat content is lower. On the other hand, if you have to consume processed food, like bread, opt for the whole grain bread as its high in dietary fiber content. Fiber assists in burning calories.

Also things to avoid are, refined sugar containing products and junk food. Look for sugar substitutes to use in the place of sugar. Junk food is low in nutritional value and high in calories content. Avoid it as well. However, ensure you consume plenty of fruits and vegetables and minimize on starch products for an almost ideal body weight.

Never Break the Law of Three.

Commit yourself to do at least three days of cardio and at least three days of either resistance training or body weight training a week. Cardio and your strength training can be on the same day if time is an issue, but never break the law of three unless you are deathly ill. This is how people stay fit for life.

Don't Poison Yourself at the Dinner Table.

After 7 weeks I'm sure you've developed a taste for healthier food. Keep your momentum going. An occasional cheat day aside, or some snacks with friends is one thing, but don't fall into eating any junk that crosses your path.

Make Fit Friends.

Positive peer pressure can be a wonderful thing. With fit friends you will feel a greater social nudge to keep yourself also moving in the direction of the fit and healthy. When the gym becomes a spot you enjoy going to socially you are making great strides towards really adopting a true fitness lifestyle!

Explore Exciting New Fitness Realms.

Keep things interesting. Why not explore yoga, Pilates or the fun and craziness of Kettlebell conditioning? Fresh fitness experiences can help motivation, be great fun and help you become more well-rounded and athletic. Ask someone who has been living a healthy lifestyle for years and I'm sure they'll have a long interesting list of fitness adventures! You should too!

Maria Garcia
Teach What You Have Learned.

A wiser man than me said the best way to keep something is to give it away. How true. Do you have a friend or loved one you could help get into shape showing them the principles you have learned? Sharing your experience is a great way to keep yourself moving in the right direction. Life can be funny like that!

ABOUT THE AUTHOR

Maria Garcia literally grew up in a gym. Her family runs a chain of gyms in Detroit. Her father is a fitness instructor while her estranged mother used to be a diet and lifestyle consultant.

When her father could no longer fulfil his duties as a fitness instructor, Maria took over. It was an easy decision since she has been exposed to the world of gyms, muscle building and fitness ever since she was young.

Today, Maria is a well-known fitness guru.